Mediterranean Diet Cookbook

70 Easy, Healthy, and Flavorful Mediterranean Recipes for Everyday Cooking

By

Jason A. Patton

© Copyright 2021 by Jason A. Patton- All rights reserved.

This document is geared towards providing exact and reliable information in regards to the topic and issue covered. The publication is sold with the idea that the publisher is not required to render accounting, officially permitted, or otherwise, qualified services. If advice is necessary, legal or professional, a practiced individual in the profession should be ordered.

- From a Declaration of Principles which was accepted and approved equally by a Committee of the American Bar Association and a Committee of Publishers and Associations.

In no way is it legal to reproduce, duplicate, or transmit any part of this document in either electronic means or in printed format. Recording of this publication is strictly prohibited and any storage of this document is not allowed unless with written permission from the publisher. All rights reserved.

The information provided herein is stated to be truthful and consistent, in that any liability, in terms of inattention or otherwise, by any usage or abuse of any policies, processes, or directions contained within is the solitary and utter responsibility of the recipient reader.

Under no circumstances will any legal responsibility or blame be held against the publisher for any reparation, damages, or monetary loss due to the information herein, either directly or indirectly.

Respective authors own all copyrights not held by the publisher.

The information herein is offered for informational purposes solely, and is universal as so. The presentation of the information is without contract or any type of guarantee assurance.

The trademarks that are used are without any consent, and the publication of the trademark is without permission or backing by the trademark owner. All trademarks and brands within this book are for clarifying purposes only and are the owned by the owners themselves, not affiliated with this document.

Table of content

INTRODUCTION THE MEDITERRANEAN DIET UP CLOSE 5

CHAPTER 1 THE 12 BASIC GUIDING PRINCIPLES OF THE MEDITERRANEAN DIET 9

CHAPTER 2 THE BENEFITS OF THE MEDITERRANEAN DIET 24

CHAPTER 3 MEDITERRANEAN DIET: TWO WEEKS WEIGHT LOSS PLAN 29

CHAPTER 4 HOW TO STOCK PANTRY AND FRIDGE ... 42

CHAPTER 5 HOW TO EAT OUT 45

CHAPTER 6 MEDITERRANEAN DIET: MAINTENANCE MEAL PLAN 48

CHAPTER 7 MEDITERRANEAN DIET: FOOD FOR KIDS 56

CHAPTER 8 RECIPES FOR MEDITERRANEAN WEIGHT LOSS DIET 63

Introduction The Mediterranean Diet Up Close

The term Mediterranean diet refers to a specific combination of foods rich in antioxidants, minerals, and vitamins together with a perfect balance of fatty acids. However, it may not be classified as one of the typical meal plans followed to achieve targeted health outcomes, especially weight loss. In fact, Mediterranean diet (MD) is not just about eating food as you cannot eat your way for weight loss or for better health. MD is actually a harmony of diet and lifestyle which results in a healthy life balance ever so elusive in practically all regions of the world except Greece, Crete, Italy and Spain. The latter regions are often geographically identified as the Mediterranean basin.

The Mediterranean diet is not merely a fad as it has been in practice since time immemorial in the region. While fad diets vanish to oblivion in just a short span of time, MD persisted through the years.

Its vaunted efficacy for a long roster of health benefits evolved from tradition and word-of-mouth to unproven claims and conjectures, until scientific research documented the link between typical food consumed by a specific population on one hand and their longevity and low prevalence of chronic and coronary diseases on the other hand. MD is the sum total of food included in the diet, how food is eaten, and how various desirable practices are synergized to create a potent life balance for healthy living.

Therefore, MD may be more appropriately referred to as the Mediterranean healthy lifestyle.

As readers would have noticed, the region where the MD originated comprises of several groups of culturally different people. However, despite marked changes in their traditional diets and comfort foods, the people in this region are aware of the importance of enjoying their meal and whenever possible, they enjoy a hearty midday meal with the whole family.

Chapter 1 presents the 12 basic guiding principles of the Mediterranean diet.

The benefits of adopting the Mediterranean diet for one's health are explained in Chapter 2. Chapter 3 introduces the reader to a special Two-Week Weight Loss Plan based on the principles of this heart-friendly diet. Meanwhile, Chapter 4 offers suggestions about how to stock the home pantry and the fridge of goodies for preparing meals the Mediterranean way. Chapter 5 presents dining out ideas for individuals or families faithfully subscribed to the Mediterranean diet.

The maintenance meal plan for the two-week weight loss initiative is bared in Chapter 6. Believing that healthy children are the happiest children, the seventh chapter of the book is dedicated to foods in the Mediterranean diet which are great for kids. Chapter 8 carries the highlight of this eBook, sumptuous recipes of dishes in the traditional tailor-fitted for the weight-loss plan using the low- carbs approach.

The Mediterranean diet food pyramid is also shown in this chapter. The recipes features dishes categorized in terms of the following: fish, dessert, legumes, meat, pasta rice bread, poultry, salad, snack, soup, and vegetables. A bonus chapter on the tips for Mediterranean cooking caps your healthy read.

Enjoy the food and stay healthy the Mediterranean way!

Chapter 1 The 12 Basic Guiding Principles of the Mediterranean Diet

Consume Lots of Fruits

There is no limit with regard to the choice of fruits to include in the MD. However, since fruits contain vitamins and nutrients in different quantities, it is always better to go with dark-colored fruits, which nutritionists claim to deliver an extra-ordinary nutritional punch. Dark-colored fruits especially the dark red and orange ones, and even vegetables provide anti-oxidants and phyto-nutrients. Variety is also an essential factor in choosing fruits for the MD.

The following fruits are commonly grown in the Mediterranean: figs, grapes, lemons, mandarin oranges, olives, persimmons, and pomegranates. Other important fruits in the MD are blackberries, blueberries, cranberries, plums, red grapes, and red raspberries. MD experts also recommend succulent or those containing lots of fiber and water, such as: apples, oranges, peaches, and watermelons. The idea behind extra water and fiber in the diet is to help weight watchers feel satisfied longer and to aid in the digestive process.

Whereas there is no limit to the choice of fruits which can be included in the diet, servings will have to be controlled. Moreover, there should be more vegetables than fruits in the diet, for two main reasons: first, fruits have more calories than vegetables; and second, fruits do not have much diversity of nutrients than vegetables. One and a half servings of fruits a day is typical in MD. The serving size of most fruits except banana is one cup. One 8-to 9-inch banana is one serving. Fruit juices or canned fruits can be substituted for raw fruits at one cup per serving, whereas one serving of dried fruits is equivalent to one-half cup

Consume Lots of Vegetables

All vegetables may be included in the MD, but people should strive to limit their intake of corn and white potatoes because of their high starch content, which in turn contribute to more calories. The following vegetables are commonly grown in the Mediterranean: artichokes, asparagus, broccoli, broccoli rabe, cabbage, eggplant, green beans, garlic, onions, and tomatoes. Dark-colored vegetables including beets, carrots, red peppers, and sweet potatoes are excellent sources of anti-oxidants and phyto-nutrients.

Likewise, eat plenty of green, leafy vegetables other than broccoli because these are also powerhouses of nutrients: bok choy, cauliflower, collards, kale, lettuce, mustard, romaine, spinach, summer and winter squash, turnip greens and zucchini.

Broccoli rabe is also known as broccoli raab or rapini. Broccoli rabe is also known as broccoli raab or rapini.

Collard is also known as non-heading cabbage or tree-cabbage Collard is also known as non-heading cabbage or tree-cabbage

Adults need to consume at least two cups of vegetables in the MD. Vegetables may be eaten raw, cooked or using them as ingredients to other dishes. For those who would like to try the MD but are hesitating because they don't like to eat a lot of vegetables would be glad to know that vegetable serving sizes do not have to be large. The following average vegetable intake requirements may serve as your guide in preparing meals the Mediterranean way. The good news is, it conforms to the dietary guidelines of health and nutrition authorities:

At least 1 ½ cups of orange-colored vegetables per week At least 2 cups per week of dark green vegetables

At least 5 ½ cups per week of other vegetables

For those trying the MD for healthy eating, at least 2 ½ cups per week of starchy vegetables, but those doing the MD for weight loss should refrain from or limit intake of starch-rich vegetables to a maximum of 1 cup in a week.

Consume Legumes

Legumes are complete in the macronutrients carbohydrates, proteins, and fats and oils, whereas fruits and vegetables do not have fats and oils. Legumes are also rich in vitamins B1, B3, B6, and B9 and in minerals such as calcium, magnesium, and molybdenum. The following legumes are commonly grown in the Mediterranean: chickpeas, lentils, and peas. However, legumes for inclusion in the MD are limitless and may also include black beans, black-eyed peas, great northern beans, kidney beans, and split beans.

For those who are not fond of eating legumes, you may choose just two and add these in your soups and stews. Legumes add a lot of flavor in food, provides your fiber needs, and have very little fat. At least 2½ cups of legumes per week are required in the MD.

Include Nuts and Seeds in your Diet

Nuts and seeds are a staple in Mediterranean cuisine, either as the main ingredient in a snack recipe or to add wonderful flavor to food. The following nuts commonly grown in the Mediterranean are: almonds, hazelnuts, pine nuts, and walnuts. Other healthy nuts and seeds that are indispensable in the MD are: Brazil nuts, cashew nuts, chia seeds, flaxseeds or linseeds, macadamia nuts, peanuts (although peanuts are really legumes), pecan nuts, pistachio nuts, pumpkin seeds, sesame seeds, and sunflower seeds. Quinoa (actually not a true cereal but a pseudocereal) may be considered a seed.

With all the great benefits which can be derived from nuts and seeds especially healthy fats, these food items also contain calories. Those who are watching their weight or are following the MD diet for weight loss should control their consumption of nuts and seeds. Here are approximate numbers of some nuts that typically comprise an ounce - the typical serving size of nuts:

- Almonds: 20 to 25

- Brazil nuts: 6 to 8

- Cashew nuts: 16 to 18

- Hazel nuts: 10 to 12

- Peanuts: 28

- Pecan nuts: 15 halves Pine nuts: 50 to 157

- Pistachios: 45 to 47

- Walnuts: 14 halves

A caveat about nuts: Brazil nuts, cashew nuts and peanuts have higher content of unhealthy fats. The best nuts are almonds and walnuts because of their Omega 3 content and their great flavor. Nuts are best when they are raw, but if you really had to cook them then go for toasted nuts. Also make sure that they are unsalted and uncoated, and with no added sugar and fat. Also, the claims about chia seeds have not yet been scientifically proven, so they must be consumed in moderate servings of one ounce at the most

Eat whole grains, especially whole grain bread

Technically, the term whole grain refers to the grain or process grain products where the caryopsis consisting of the anatomical components bran, germ and endosperm are intact whether they are ground, cracked, or flaked. Whole grains are integral to the MD as they contain high amounts of fiber and impart natural goodness to food. Among the whole grain produce common in the Mediterranean region are: barley, corn, rice, and wheat. If you love bread, choose dense, heavy chewy breads baked from while wheat, barley, and oats. If you love pasta, choose whole grain pasta products from the supermarket.

There are many reasons for choosing whole grain foods not only for their health benefits but also for that feeling of fullness you need for your daily routines. MD experts also recommend steel-cut, whole-grain oatmeal and multi-grain hot cereals. The good news with MD is that it allows people a wide choice of whole grains. Even those who love rice can enjoy eating rice as long as they chose brown rice. Couscous and polenta are also excellent whole grain choices.

Whole grains are an integral part of the Mediterraneandiet. Whole grains are an integral part of the Mediterranean diet.

Use Olive Oil in Cooking and in Salads

Olive oil is the main fat source used in the MD. Thus, the consumption of olive oil in Mediterranean countries is high even of other less expensive oils are becoming popular. With the current interest in MD, even non-Mediterranean countries such as Germany, Japan, UK and US have increasing consumption of olive oil. Olive oil defines the distinctive flavor of the MD and is therefore of particular significance in the overall context of the MD.

Olive oil not only increases the palatability of foods but also improves the texture and enhances the flavor. In Greece, the very popular lathera dish contains vegetables cooked in an olive oil-based sauce, tomatoes, and garlic. Leading authorities on the MD believes that without using olive oil in the preparation of Mediterranean dishes, it would be practically impossible for people in Greece and in the surrounding countries in the region to consume high quantities of vegetables and legumes.

Olive oil is used in the Mediterranean diet not only for cooking but also for the following purposes among others:

Raw olive oil is used in aiolli and other dips; Vegetable marinades;

Flavoring for soups and stews by long, slow cooking, especially in

pistou;

For batter, dough, and several pastries;

Bread with oil, which is considered as elemental Mediterranean cuisine, such as the Catalan dish pa amb oli.

Mediterranean people very rarely use butter in their cuisine and they do not miss it because olive oil has its basic appeal for their dishes. In occasions where olive oil does not suit a particular recipe, canola oil is used instead. Extra virgin olive oil, particularly the lighter version is the best choice for salad dressings, for use in foods eaten raw, and in baking. However, for cooking, regular extra virgin oil available in the supermarket is just fine. One should not hesitate to prepare foods the Mediterranean way because of the cost of olive oil since it will replace butter and margarine. The small cost added in using olive is nothing compared to its health benefits.

Include Moderate Amounts of Low Fat Dairy or If Possible, Non-Fat Dairy

In the Mediterranean, goat and sheep milk are more preferred than cow's milk. However, as long as you choose low-fat or non-fat milk, it is good enough for inclusion in the MD. Rather than the usual Western cheese, yogurt is a very important constituent of the MD, together with some hard and soft varieties of cheese. Greek yogurt has a rich silky texture and is widely available in many supermarkets in the US. It is a better choice because it has two times the protein content of regular commercial yogurt but costs the same as the name-brand regular yogurt.

There is even fat-free Greek yogurt for weight-watchers which is already available in the US. Even Starbucks has jumped into the Greek yogurt bandwagon and is teaming up with a Greek yogurt manufacturer.

By next year, Americans hooked up with the healthy Mediterranean diet can buy ready-to-eat Greek yogurt parfaits from the multi-chain international coffee store.

Meanwhile, the MD is not known for its heavy use of cheese. Rather, cheese is used more as a flavoring to enhance the flavor of food, but not necessarily to overwhelm it. Cheese is also used in MD in combination with dessert. If you like cheese, make sure that it is also the low-fat variety and consume dairy products in moderation.

Eat Fish and Shellfish

Influenced by geography, the Mediterranean diet includes seafood as one of its integral components. Moreover, the selection of fish in the traditional diet is largely responsible for the heart-healthy reputation of the MD diet. Fish like cod, haddock, mackerel, red mullet, salmon, and sardines, which are cold-water fish varieties, are rich in Omega 3 and other unsaturated fats. Squid and octopus are also staple seafood in the MD. Consuming fish with high Omega 3 instead of animal meats ensures that the body's arteries are not clogged and are protected from coronary diseases.

Other fish not necessary from the Mediterranean which are rich in Omega 3 and unsaturated fats are Albacore tuna, anchovies, Arctic char or iwana, Atlantic mackerel, sablefish or black cod, Pacific halibut, rainbow trout, shad, smelt, and wild salmon. Shellfish are also welcome in the MD. Among the healthiest are clams, crab, lobster, mussels, oysters, scallops, and shrimps.

Include the Right (Healthy) Fats in your Diet

Not all fats are bad for one's health. In fact, most people who observe and/or read about the MD see that Mediterranean people do not necessarily consume a low-fat diet. However, research evidence such as the findings of the study conducted by the Keys husband-and-wife team showed that these people have healthy heart conditions. The explanation for this phenomenon lies in the consumption of healthier types of fats such as monounsaturated fats and polyunsaturated omega 3 fatty acids. These are the right kinds of fat that should be included in the diet.

Make Physical Activity Part of your Daily Routine

A good dose of daily physical activity is part of the Mediterranean lifestyle. The MD will not be as effective as it is for people who do not like to indulge in physical activity in exercise on a regular basis. The rural folks from the Mediterranean region do not care about doing aerobics or cardio exercises.

However, they have plenty of daily physical activity through the work they engage in, traveling where they needed to go on foot, and having fun. Modern living in any part of the world may not always allow people to do what the Mediterranean folks do, but they can benefit from the MD by working out, doing aerobic exercises, and engaging in strength training exercises

Drink Wine in Moderate Amounts

Red wine is recommended, but not a "must" in the Mediterranean diet. It provides protection to the heart from the anti-oxidants from flavonoids in the skin of the grapes.

Flavonoids lower the risk of heart disease because it lowers bad cholesterol, increases good cholesterol, and reduces blood clotting in the arteries.

Studies are now underway to verify another health benefit from the flavonoid called resveratrol, also found in red wine. It is claimed that resveratrol inhibits tumor development in certain cancers.

In place of red wine for those who do not drink alcoholic beverages, grape juice manufactured from Concord grapes work just as fine. Likewise, eating purple grapes also offers the same benefits for a healthy heart. As a matter of precaution, however, the recommended daily intake in conjunction with the MD is four ounces daily for women and two four-ounce intakes for men. Like any other food, anything consumed in excess affects the health negatively. Excessive drinking even of red wine will result in hypertension, cardiovascular conditions, and excess calories.

Red wine in the MD is recommended only for individuals who are in good health. Never consume alcohol if you have been prescribed a daily dose of aspirin for a medical condition. If you have any of the following conditions, you are not to drink any alcoholic beverages as doing so will cause your condition to worsen:

- Congestive heart failure; High triglycerides level
- Hypertension (high blood pressure); Liver disease; and/or
- Pancreatitis.

- Eat Very Small Servings of
- Red Meat Occasionally

In the Mediterranean diet, red meat is consumed rarely, as in only once or twice a week. However, for clarity, the servings should be limited. If you want to have red meat twice a week, make sure you consume no more than a total of 12 ounces for the week. Lean cuts should be consumed, which suggests that the fat portion needs to be trimmed out. If you use red meat as ingredient to soup or pasta, this should be counted as part of the 12 ounces limit per week.

People may feel that they are severely restricted in their red meat consumption. They are right. However, the restriction is necessary because red meat is a major contributing factor to cancer, heart disease, and stroke. After all, you do not embark on a Mediterranean diet just to savor the delectable cuisine of the region. You are doing it for your health.

Chapter 2 The Benefits of the Mediterranean Diet

In the groundbreaking Seven Countries Study of the 1950s conducted by Ancel and Margaret Keys, results confirmed the association between the kind of food people eat on one hand, and life expectancy and the prevalence of chronic and coronary diseases on the other hand. The study was conducted in the Mediterranean region. The findings verified that consumption of food notably low in fat leads to higher life expectancy and very low prevalence of chronic diseases, particularly chronic heart disease. From thereon, interest was focused on the beneficial effects of the Mediterranean diet. This marked the origin of the concept of the Mediterranean diet (MD).

Based on the discussion in Chapter 1, readers will not definitely associate MD with a vegetarian or vegan diet. With fish, meat, and dairy components, the MD is delightfully flavorful and abounds in hedonistic qualities.

Yet, the diets were frugal and do not have excessive calories.

Adding up to the moderate calorie intake is regular physical activity, though not exactly the idea of physical activity popular in the gyms of Western countries, but extensive enough to result in lower rates of obesity in the Mediterranean region. Thus, the healthy Mediterranean lifestyle was thought to be something good to emulate.

Further studies later buttressed the Keys' findings and a roster of health benefits had been compiled. In no time, a new and effective regimen for health and longevity was born. This chapter summarizes the beneficial effects of the Mediterranean diet. Results of three recent studies showed that:

From a study published in the British Medical Journal in the year 2008, following the traditional MD resulted in a 9% decreased in deaths from coronary artery disease.

In 2011, a systematic review published in the Journal of the American College of Cardiology involving 535,000 cases revealed that

traditional MD is correlated with lower blood pressure, and lower levels blood glucose and triglycerides.

In early 2013, a study among 7,447 cases of high risk of cardiovascular conditions showed no significant difference among three groups in the reduction of risk for heart attack, stroke, and heart disease. Two groups both followed the traditional MD but one group was supplemented with olive, while the other was supplement with nuts. The third group followed a low-fat diet.

As compiled by Denver physician Eric Zacharias in 2012, MD is effective in the prevention of obesity and in weight loss. From the same compilation, Dr.

Zacharias also noted that the MD is associated with reduced overall mortality rate and reduced risk for a number of medical conditions including:

- Allergic rhinitis Alzheimer's disease Arthritis
- Asthma Atopy Cancer
- Cardiovascular diseases Dementia
- Depression
- Macular degeneration (age-related) Metabolic syndrome
- Parkinson's disease Rheumatoid arthritis Type 2 diabetes

Other health benefits of the MD with respect to better quality of life include: Healthy aging

Healthy vision Improved memory Strong bones and teeth

Stronger immune system

Chapter 3 Mediterranean Diet: Two Weeks Weight Loss Plan

Week 1 Weight Loss Plan Day 1: Sunday Breakfast Grape Juice

Chickpea and Barley Glee Fruit in season or pear

Morning Snack

Pumpkin seeds

Lunch

Lamb Loin Chops

Fruit in season or orange Red wine or cranberry juice

Afternoon Snack

Frutti Smoothie No. 1

Dinner

Baked Salmon with Honey-Balsamic Glaze Fruit in season

Red wine or apple juice (if you had red wine for lunch have apple juice or any other MD fruit recommendations for dinner)

Day 2: Monday Breakfast

Lemon Juice

Apple-Walnut Delight

Fruit in season or persimmon

Morning Snack

Quinoa

Lunch

Salmon-Asparagus Omelet (Frittata) Fruit in season or plums

Red wine or orange juice

Afternoon Snack

Frutti Smoothie No. 2

Dinner

Broiled halibut

Fruit in season or peaches

Red wine or orange juice (if you had red wine for lunch have orange juice or any other MD fruit recommendations for dinner)

Day 3: Tuesday Breakfast

Non-fat goat's milk Breakfast Rush Fruit in season

Morning Snack

Flaxseeds

Lunch

Sesame Tuna Temptation Fruit in season

Four seasons natural juice (homemade, juice four of your favorite fruits and drink)

Afternoon Snack

Frutti Smoothie No. 3

Dinner

Grilled Shrimp Fruit in season Red wine punch

Day 4: Wednesday Breakfast

Breakfast Rush Fruit in season

Morning Snack

Snack Pack (half of the serving for breakfast, see recipe on Chapter 8 for Breakfast Rush.)

Lunch

Sesame Tuna Temptation Fruit in season

Pineapple juice

Afternoon Snack

Frutti Smoothie No. 4

Dinner

Steamed Oysters Fruit in season Fruit punch

Day 5: Thursday Breakfast

Fruit Salad Mediterranean Style Brown Rice and Stuffed Chicken Carrot Soup

Morning Snack

Chia seeds

Lunch

Lentil soup Fruit in season

Chili Chicken and Beans

Afternoon Snack

Savory Mixed Nuts

Dinner

Lime Chicken Fruit in season

Celery and fennel soup

Day 6: Friday Breakfast

Hot Lemon and Honey Walnut Baklava

Fruit in season Morning Snack

Frutti Smoothie 5

Lunch

Fish Stew in Saffron and White Beans Fruit in season

Red wine

Afternoon Snack

Walnut Baklava (half serving)

Dinner

Grouper in Tomato-Olive Sauce Eggplant and Tomato Pesto Turkey Soup

Day 7: Saturday Breakfast

Non-fat milk

Mixed Vegetable Omelet Fruit in season

Morning Snack

Lunch

Mixed nuts and seeds (1/2 cup)

Salmon and Cashew Fruit in season Tomato soup

Afternoon Snack

Frutti Smoothie 3

Dinner

Fennel, White Beans and Seared Salmon Frutti Smoothie No. 6

Green soup

Week 2 Weight Loss Plan Day 1: Sunday Breakfast Frutti Smoothie No. 6

Bean and sausage soup Poached fish

Morning Snack

Pistachios and pecan nuts

Lunch

Fish curry and vegetables Fruit in season Minestrone soup

Afternoon Snack

Frutti Smoothie No. 7

Dinner

Zucchini Gratin Fruit in season

Fish and Seafood Primavera

Day 2: Monday Breakfast

Rice Pudding

Pepper and Red Snapper Fruit in season

Morning Snack

Almonds or walnuts

Lunch

Ground Round Special Ala Turk Lettuce and cucumber salad

Red wine or orange juice

Afternoon Snack

Banana

Dinner

Tuna Casserole

Fruit in season or peaches Pumpkin and sweet potato soup

Day 3: Tuesday Breakfast

Whole grain oats (rolled) Non-fat or skim milk Fruit in season

Morning Snack

A little Feta cheese and whole grain bread

Lunch

Roasted Vegetable Chowder Fruit Salad Mediterranean-Style Mediterranean Tuna

Afternoon Snack

Apples and grapes

Dinner

Grilled Mediterranean Seafood with S-dip Fruit in season

Potato Leek Soup

Day 4: Wednesday Breakfast

Mediterranean Toast Frutti Smoothie No. 8 Apple juice

Morning Snack

Quinoa salad

Lunch

Chicken Chili Fruit in season Pea soup

Afternoon Snack

Cucumber in natural sweetened vinegar

Dinner

Pasta and Sardines Frutti Smoothie No. 9 Cabbage soup

Red wine

Day 5: Thursday Breakfast

Greek salad Grape juice Grilled seafood

Morning Snack

Soy milk

Lunch

Marinated mushroom Fruit in season or orange

Mediterranean salmon or tuna

Afternoon Snack

Frutti Smoothie No. 9

Dinner

Stuffed Tomatoes Shrimp and pasta Red wine

Day 6: Friday Breakfast

Sugar-free gelato

Mediterranean low-cholesterol pizza Fruit in season

Morning Snack

Peaches

Lunch

Greek seafood burger Fruit in season Orange juice

Afternoon Snack

Frutti Smoothie No. 10

Dinner

Stuffed Pepper Roast Fruit in season

Bourbon-glazed tuna or salmon Kale and chicken soup

Day 7: Saturday Breakfast

Pumpkin and corn muffin Fruit in season

Walnut milk Morning Snack

Quinoa light salad

Lunch

Mediterranean seafood stew Fruit in season

Pasta and shrimps

Afternoon Snack

Pumpkin and corn muffin

Dinner

Grilled Vegetable salad Fruit in season Poached shellfish

Red wine punch

Chapter 4 How to Stock Pantry and Fridge

The Mediterranean diet emphasizes the use of fresh food items instead of processed (i.e., canned) products if this can be helped. However, there are a few staples which need to be kept at hand in the fridge or in the pantry. Many convenience meals and snacks for the diet had to be kept cold. Fresh produce can be kept in a fridge.

Stuff for the Refrigerator and Freezer

Following are the basic items which individuals or families following the Mediterranean diet regimen should always have ready in the fridge:

Bread and rolls; Carton of eggs;

Fresh vegetables, including carrots, celery, and lettuce; Honey or maple syrup;

Cheese (sourced from goat or sheep); Greek yogurt, both regular and low-fat; 1-percent milk or cottage cheese;

Nuts

Natural nut butters such as peanuts and almond butter Condiments including Cayenne or Tabasco sauce, mustard sauce, Worcestershire sauce, salsas, and mayonnaise.

Weekly food supplies from the supermarket such as fish, chicken, and meat should always be kept in the freezer. Frozen products such as frozen berries, frozen vegetables, and frozen shrimps should also be kept in the freezer right after shopping.

Meanwhile, minced garlic and minced ginger should be kept in the refrigerator. For bigger amounts of minced garlic, the freezer presents a better storage option.

Stuff for the Pantry

The following seasonings may be stored in the pantry using an airtight container: Brown sugar

- Chili powder Cinnamon Curry powder Cumin
- Italian seasoning

- Low-sodium soy sauce Pepper

- Salt Vinegar

Olive oil, canola oil, and cooking spray are usually stocked in the pantry shelf. Likewise, cooking ingredients packed in boxes, cans, and jars are stocked in the pantry shelves or drawers. Keep the following handy in your pantry:

Black beans Brown rice Bulgur Chickpeas Diced tomatoes

Dried fruits: apricots, raisins, etc.

Dried lentils Light tuna chunks Oatmeal

Seeds; flaxseed, pumpkin, sunflower Spaghetti sauce

Whole grain pasta

Cooking wines (unopened) such as white and red wine, balsamic vinegar, etc.

Chapter 5 How to Eat Out

Fortunately, the Mediterranean diet is not a very restrictive meal that eating out while you're on this diet would be a big challenge, if not totally impossible. You can even drink red wine. The main food restrictions you are to remember when dining out are red meat, high-fat dairy, and refined grains. There are lots of restaurants which offer delectable vegetable and seafood dishes in their menu.

With emerging technology, you can even surf the net for restaurants serving Mediterranean cuisine and look at their menu.

When you eat out, the greatest danger of spoiling any gains you have achieved from following the MD is exceeding your calories and over-eating. Restaurant servings are traditionally bigger than the ones we have at home, most especially if you are the one preparing your MD. It wouldn't hurt to prepare a list of the maximum amount of food items you can still include in your dine-out meal.

Limit the portion of the servings you consume.

Call the restaurant where you plan to dine out and ask questions about how their dishes are prepared. It is your right to know these things as a consumer. If you are fond of pasta, you can ask if they are using whole grain pasta. If they don't, you can make a request for a special meal of whole grain pasta. The sauce need not be pork or beef since there are restaurants who serve spaghetti in tuna sauce. You can also request that instead of using butter or animal fats or oil with trans fats, use extra virgin olive oil. Special arrangements can always be made with restaurants especially if you are a regular. Opt not to have cheese in your pasta.

Dining out means socializing with other people. Make sure to enjoy eating your food with your friends and family and eat very slowly. As your serving is expected to be more than the typical MD serving, you can always set aside the appropriate portion that you need and have the waiter pack the rest "to go" before you even start eating. Perhaps, if another member of your family is also on the MD, you can share meals.

Order a fish dish instead of red meat, pork or chicken. Select dishes which are not prepared using too much oil or butter. The manner of food preparation will serve as clues to the oil/fat content of the dish. Opt for broiled or grilled dishes, as well as seared or steamed ones. if your friends are amenable, you can dine out in Mediterranean restaurants. There must be a couple or more of such restaurants in your city.

Dining out is not really a problem for people who adopted the Mediterranean diet in their lifestyle. Dining out is not really a problem for people who adopted the Mediterranean diet in their lifestyle.

Chapter 6 Mediterranean Diet: Maintenance Meal Plan

Reality Check

Some individuals embark on a diet regimen as part of a weight loss goal. This is exactly the objective for writing this eBook. However, anybody who dreams of losing weight using the MD or any other diet plan should be in synch with reality. If you gained weight over the course of several weeks to a month due to low physical activity and/or eating more than your body's energy requirements, you would have packed between 5 to 7 pounds. This book's two-week weight loss plan in Chapter 3 plus enough exercise and sunshine will certainly be very effective for your target weight goal.

While medical practitioners and other experts do not have a single consensus on the safe weight loss rate, the safest number is in the range of one half to two pounds in a week. Therefore, if your goal is to lose 7 pounds in two weeks, that would be fairly safe. If you have packed in 30 pounds over the course of two to three years, that is a different story.

If you go down by one pound over the course of two weeks, you lost weight safety and normally. If you lost 4 to 6 pounds in two weeks, rejoice! You have done very well. Yet whether you are in the first or second case, you have not lost all the 30 pounds yet in the aforementioned example. That is what this chapter is for. In fact, even the case mentioned in the first paragraph needs to go through Chapter 7 - the maintenance plan.

For the purpose of the maintenance plan, individuals whose goal is 7 pounds or less of weight loss have been achieved will be called Case A, whereas those whose goal is over 7 pounds of weight loss or those who have not attained their

target weight loss goals will be called Case B. Separate maintenance plans are drawn for the two cases.

Maintenance Plan: Case A-Target Weight Achieved in 2 Weeks

1. For those who have achieved their target weight within 2 weeks, the following week (third week) is the transition towards the maintenance phase. In the transition phase, one will decide whether to put in more carbs or more variety of carbs in his/her MD (Plan A) or continue with the usual low-carbs intake of the MD for the previous two weeks (Plan S; S for status quo or no change).

1. In Plan A, the maintenance plan is to slightly increase carbs intake, either by increasing the serving to a half of the previous two weeks but using the same carbohydrate constituents of the two-week plan or having more leeway. For example, instead of lower-calorie brown rice cakes for the Greek pita recipe, the real pita may be used. One has the free choice of any of the recipes provided in Chapter 8.

1. As the term status quo suggests, Plan S will retain the same low-carbs approach as in the previous two weeks. One may choose any from the recipes in Chapter 8 except for the Pasta Bread Rice category.

1. After the third week, weights are checked again. If those who used Plan A either continued losing their weight as in the two-week plan or maintained their achieved target weight, they can use Plan A as their regular maintenance plan.

1. Those who used Plan S and continued losing their weight as in the two-week plan or maintained their achieved target weight can now use Plan A as their maintenance plan.

1. Repeat steps 4 or 5 as the case may be for the fourth week.

1. If those who chose Plan A or Plan S start to gain weight after a week of the plan, revert back to the two-week MD weight loss plan.

1. After two weeks, follow the same steps of this maintenance plan.

1. It will do no harm if you decide to continue longer with the maintenance plan unless you experience alarming weight loss rate, which is very unlikely.

Maintenance Plan: Case B - Target Weight Not Achieved in 2 Weeks

1. For those who have not achieved their target weight within 2 weeks, the following week (third week) is the start of the maintenance plan.

1. For simplicity and convenience, one mixes and matches his/her favorite menu form the low-carbs MD diet during the first two weeks. The rules are simple:

a. Foods for breakfast from the schedule in Chapter 3 may be used for breakfast lunch or dinner, but not for snack.

b. The same rule applies for lunch and dinner foods.

c. Snack foods from the schedule in Chapter 3 may only be used as snack.

d. If you want to try any of the recipes in Chapter 8, please feel free to do so.

1. After the third week, weights are checked again. Those who either continued losing their weight as in the two-week can use Plan A from Case A as their regular maintenance plan. Going over Plan A, the maintenance plan is to slightly increase carbs intake, either by increasing the serving to a half of the previous two weeks but using the same carbohydrate constituents of the two-week plan or having more leeway. For example, instead of lower-calorie brown rice cakes for the Greek pita recipe, the real pita may be used. One has the free choice of any of the recipes provided in Chapter 8.

1. For those who gained weight during the third week, use step 2 above as your maintenance plan.

1. Repeat steps 3 or 4 as the case may be for the fourth week.

1. Those who start to gain weight after the fourth week of the plan, revert back to the two-weight MD weight loss plan.

1. After two weeks, follow the same steps of this maintenance plan.

1. Repeat the cycle until you have reached your ideal weight.

1.   It will do no harm if you decide to continue longer with the maintenance plan unless you experience alarming weight loss rate, which is very unlikely.

Alternately, after you have achieved your ideal weight, you may be interested to eat more of the plant-based foods discussed in this book. You can experiment with your own recipes, but limit your ingredients to the foods mentioned in Chapter 2 and those used in the recipes in Chapter 8. Also, as part of your long term weight maintenance plan, eating more fruits and vegetables had been linked

with lower prevalence of cancer, coronary heart disease, and stroke.

Moreover, in many weight loss program, regular physical activity is a must. Diet alone cannot maintain a healthy weight. You have to burn the calories you take in when you eat or drink. Exercise every day.

Your battle with the scale and the tape measure will gain ground with the Mediterranean diet.

Your battle with the scale and the tape measure will gain ground with the Mediterranean diet.

Chapter 7 Mediterranean Diet: Food for Kids

At this point in your reading, you may be wondering if children will also grow healthy with a Mediterranean diet. The decision is easier for other older members of the family because it will be more convenient to prepare the MD diet if everyone or almost everyone is into it. Here are some statistics which might help you decide whether or not to train children earlier for the Mediterranean lifestyle:

One of every 400 children and adolescents in the US suffers from diabetes.

More than a quarter of Americans less than 20 years of age, which translate to 215,000 young people have diabetes.

Over one third of children and adolescents in the US are either obese or overweight;

Over the past three decades, the prevalence of childhood obesity in the US has doubled;

Seven in every 10 obese youth develop at least one risk factor for heart disease.

Obese adolescents tend to develop to pre-diabetes or high blood sugar levels, which heightens the risk of diabetes.

Now that the picture is clearer, nobody would want their children to continue with the modern American kid's diet of hamburgers, fries, chocolates, and too many sweets. It is never early for young children to be introduced to the heart- healthy lifestyle of the kiddie Mediterranean diet. Carbohydrates-containing food is most frequently consumed by both adults and children. Training children to eat healthy means teaching them to eat plant starches which are the most important carbohydrates of the diet. Plant starches are found in the produce section of grocery stores and supermarkets, mainly from fresh fruits and vegetables.

With the surge of obesity and diabetes rates among children, parents have to educate children about foods that will affect their glycemic index (GI). This index is a measure of how much the blood sugar increases in a given period after consuming at least 50 grams of carbohydrates.

When children eat high GI foods, the pancreas tend to produce excessive amounts of insulin. This, in turn results in the deposition of fat in cells which put children at risk for various diseases, including cardiovascular conditions.

Even if carbs and sugar intake among children should be controlled, parents cannot keep their children on low-fat diet because it is unhealthy to do so and will most likely stunt their growth. However, children should be exposed to the good fats, fats from plants and from fish and other seafood. Olive oil and other monosaturated fat will help keep the children's heart healthy and minimize the risk of obesity and cardiovascular diseases. Moreover, children's diet should contain quality protein.

The following tables present what proteins, carbohydrates and fats should be consumed by children in the Mediterranean diet and those which should not be eaten.

Table 1: List of carbohydrates which should be eaten by children vis a vis those which they should avoid.

CONSUME or EMPHASIZE THESE CARBOHYDRATES   AVOID or LIMIT CONSUMPTION OF THESE CARBOHYDRATES

Brown rice   Anything with high sugar content

Dry beans   Cakes

Fruits: apples, bananas, blueberries, peaches, pears, strawberries Cereals in boxes (Select high-fiber or natural cereals)

Green vegetables

Whole grain bread

Whole oatmeal

Yams, sweet potatoes

Table 2: List of fats which should be included in children's diet vis a vis those which they should avoid.

CONSUME or EMPHASIZE THESE GOOD FATS   AVOID or LIMIT CONSUMPTION OF THESE UNHEALTHY FATS

- Almonds   Butter
- Cashew nuts Fats from cold cuts

- Fish oils (DHA and EPA)   Fatty meats
- Macadamia nuts   Fats from fried foods
- Peanuts
- Unprocessed peanut butter
- Walnuts

Table 3: List of proteins which should be included in children's diet vis a vis

those which they should avoid.

CONSUME or EMPHASIZE THESE PROTEINS   AVOID or LIMIT CONSUMPTION OF THESE UNHEALTHY PROTEINS

- Broiled or baked fish   Fatty beef cuts and ground beef
- Eggs   Cold cuts and lunch meats
- Lean beef   Fried protein foods
- Milk proteins: whey and casein
- Skim milk
- Skinless chicken, turkey breast

- Soy

Table 4 illustrates the foods which have low, moderate, and high glycemic index. Children had to be proper educated about foods and their corresponding category based on glycemic index so that they can hold on with the Mediterranean diet even when they are in school. Packing snacks for the kids will diminish the chance of buying unhealthy food when they are not under the watchful eyes of their parents.

Table 4. Examples of foods with low, moderate and high GI.

CONSUME or EMPHASIZE   CONSUME MODERATELY   LIMIT or AVOID CONSUMPTION

- Low GI   Moderate GI   High GI
- (GI below 50) (GI from 50 to 75)   (GI over 75)
- Apple   Balance Bar   Cakes
- Butter   Banana   Carrots
- Fructose   Brown rice   Cookies
- Grapes   Corn   Cornflakes
- Lentils   Mixed-grain breads   Glucose

- Low-carb bars   Oatmeal   High-carb bars

- Meat (lean) Potato chips Potatoes

- Milk   Table sugar   Pretzels

- Navy beans Sweet potatoes   Raisins

- Peanuts   Salted crackers

- Pinto beans   Shredded wheat

- Protein-enriched pasta   White bread

- Soy   White rice

Healthy children are happy children. Guide them through the Mediterranean diet now. It is never too

early to care for their health.

Healthy children are happy children. Guide them through the Mediterranean diet now. It is never too early to care for their health.

Chapter 8 Recipes for Mediterranean Weight Loss Diet

Here are the most sumptuous weight loss recipes of the Mediterranean diet. They taste so yummy good you won't even notice your trying to shed off pounds. Try them in your kitchen with the bonus chapter on tips for successful Mediterranean cooking. For each recipe, a code in the form 4S/BLD, which indicates:

S just before the slash indicates servings and the number before S is the number of servings.

BLD after the slash indicates breakfast, lunch, or dinner. If S is seen after the slash, it indicates that the food may also be consumed as snack food.

Fish

Salmon-Asparagus Omelet (Frittata) 4S /BLD

Sumptuous but healthy smoked salmon and asparagus frittata cooked the traditional Mediterranean way. Sumptuous but healthy smoked salmon and asparagus frittata cooked the traditional Mediterranean way.

Ingredients:

- Quantity   Measure   Food Item
- 2   tbsp. (10 ml.) Dried dill
- 1   cup (250 ml.) Egg white or egg substitute
- 0.25   tbsp. (1.25 ml.)   Ground black pepper
- 2   tbsp. (30 ml.) Extra virgin olive oil
- 0.25   cup (60 ml.)   Feta cheese (crumbled fine)
- 0.25   tbsp. (1.25 ml.)   Sea salt or kosher salt to taste (Note: May be
- lessened especially if the salmon is salty or as preferred)
- 0.25   pound (115 g.)   Sliced salmon (smoked)
- 1   pound (450 g.)   Stalks of asparagus cut in 1 in. or 2.5 cm. pieces
- 0.5   tbsp. (2.5 ml.)Tarragon

Directions:

1. Put asparagus and olive oil in a medium size ovenproof skillet and heat for 3 minutes or until the stalks soften. Add dill, pepper, salt and tarragon. Stir gently for a minute.

1. Put in the eggs in the above mixture followed immediately by the salmon and feta cheese which should be evenly distributed. Cook until the eggs are firm without covering the skillet.

1. Remove from heat and place skillet on the oven rack approximately 6 inches under the broiler. Broil the ingredients from 3 to 5 minutes or until top of the egg turns brownish.

1. Remove from broiler and serve.

Baked Salmon with Honey-Balsamic Glaze

4S/BLD (Note: Salmon may be replaced with halibut)
Ingredients:

Quantity	Measure	Food Item
4	tbsp. (60 ml.)	Balsamic vinegar
1	tbsp. (15 ml.)	Dijon mustard
3	cloves	Garlic (minced)
1	tbsp. (15 ml.)	Honey
2	tbsp.	Oregano (fresh, chopped)
0.25	tbsp. (1.25 ml.)	Ground black pepper
4	4 ounces	Salmon filets
0.25	tbsp. (1.25 ml.)	Salt to taste
1	tbsp. (15 ml.)	White wine

Directions:

1. Routine baking preparation procedure: Line baking sheet with aluminum foil; spray with canola oil cooking spray (usually PAM cooking spray); preheat oven to 400 °F.

1. Put salt and pepper on salmon filets.

1. Glaze preparation procedure:

a.   Coat a small sauce pan with cooking spray or a little canola oil.

b.   Sauté garlic in medium heat for 3 minutes or until it is soft.

c.   Mix honey, mustard, salt, vinegar and wine. Add to the cooked garlic.

d.   Simmer without cover in medium or low heat for 3 minutes or

until the glaze slightly thickens.

e.   Remove from heat and set aside half of the glaze in another container.

1.   Baking procedure for the salmon:

a.   Arrange the salmon on the baking sheet with the skin-side down.

b. Brush each piece of salmon with the remaining glaze in the saucepan.

c. Sprinkle the glazed salmon with oregano on top.

d. Bake for about 10 minutes or until salmon flakes easily with a fork.

e. Transfer the fish to plates using a turner, but leave the skin on the foil.

f. Brush the baked salmon with the glaze set aside earlier

Sesame Tuna Temptation

6S/BLD (Note: Traditionally, this recipe is called Tuna Carpaccio, an appetizer, but in a weight loss plan, this is already a full meal when a cup or less of fruits in season is consumed after this course. For lower carbohydrate content, plain rice cakes prepared from brown rice was substituted for the pita bread.)

Ingredients:

Quantity	**Measure**	**Food Item**
1	piece	Apple

1   tbsp. Ginger (fresh, minced)

3   cloves Garlic (minced)

6   pieces Rice cakes (plain, from brown rice)

1   bunch Scallions

1   tbsp. (15 ml.) Sesame oil

0.25   cup (60 ml.) Sesame seeds

0.25   tbsp. (1.25 ml.)   Soy sauce

1

Directions: pound Tuna steak (fresh)

1. Mix ginger, garlic, sesame oil and seeds, and soy well. Encrust the tuna in the mixture.

2. Heat a sauté pan to the highest level and pan-sear the tuna.

3. Add the seared tuna and the scallions to the sauce mixture.

4. Garnish with quartered apple.

5. Eat the dish with the plain rice cakes

Dessert

Apple-Walnut Delight 6S/BLDS

Ingredients:

- Quantity   Measure   Food Item
- 4   pieces Apples (medium, Rome or Gala variety, and diced into ¼ inch cubes
- 8   pieces Apricots (dried)
- 2   tbsp. Honey

- 1 tbsp. Olive oil
- ½ piece Orange (use juice and zest)
- ½ cup Walnuts (toasted and chopped

Directions:

1. Whisk the orange juice and zest, together with honey and olive oil in a salad serving bowl.

2. Add the apples and apricots. Toss these 2 fruits to coat then with the mixture in Step 1.

3. Add the chopped walnuts, toss and serve.

Fruit Salad Mediterranean Style 6S/BLDS

Ingredients:

- Quantity   Measure   Food Item

- ½ cup Almonds (toasted and chopped)
- 4 pieces Fuyu persimmons (sliced into 10 wedges)
- 1 ½ cups Grapes (cut into halves)
- 1 tbsp. Honey
- 1 tbsp. Lemon Juice
- 8 pieces Mints leaves (rolled and sliced thinly)

Directions:

1. Combine all the ingredients in a salad serving bowl.

1. Toss and serve.

1. Legumes
2. Chickpea and Barley Glee

3. 6S/BLDS

Ingredients:

- Quantity   Measure   Food Item

- 1   cup   Apricots (diced, dried)
- ¼   tsp.   Cardamom
- 1   cup   Chicken broth or as an alternative, vegetable broth
- ½   tsp.   Cinnamon
- ½   tsp.   Ginger
- 1   dash   Hot sauce
- 2   pieces   Lemon (juice and zest)
- ¼   cup   Olive oil
- 1   cup   Parsley (discard the stems and chop finely)
- ½   cup   Pearl barley
- ¼   tsp.   Pepper
- 1   cup   Pistachio nuts (shelled)
- 1   piece   Red onion (thinly sliced)
  - pinch   Salt to taste
- 8   cups   Spinach (baby spinach) leaves

- ¼ tsp. Turmeric

Directions:

1. Put the broth in a small sauce pan. Bring the broth to a boil using high heat. Add the pearl barley and cover. Remove the pan from the heat and set aside for 15 minutes.

1. Combine the apricots, chickpeas, lemon juice and zest, olive oil. parsley, red onion, and the spices in a mixing bowl. Put in the hot sauce and salt to taste.
2. Garnish by arranging the baby spinach leaves on a serving platter. Add the chickpeas and barley mixture on top of the leaves.

1. Top the salad meal with pistachios and serve.

Meat

Lamb Loin Chops 4S/LD

Ingredients:

Quantity   Measure   Food Item

- ½ cup couscous (prepared from whole wheat grains)
- 1 piece Cucumber (medium, peeled, chopped)
- 2 tbsp. Dill (fresh and finely chopped)
- ½ cup Feta cheese (crumbled)
- 1 tbsp. Garlic (minced)
- 2 pounds (or 8 pcs) Lemon juice
- 1 tbsp. Parsley (fresh and finely chopped)
- 2 tbsp. Olive oil (extra virgin)
- ¼ tsp. Salt
- 2 pieces Tomatoes (medium, chopped)
- 1 cup Water

Directions:

1. Boil water in a medium-size sauce pan.

2. To prepare the couscous:

3. a. Stir in the couscous into the boiling water from Step 1.

4. b. Bring to a boil and reduce heat just to simmer, cover the pan,

5. and wait for 5 minutes.

6. c. Use fork to fluff the simmering couscous-water mix.

7. d. Transfer to mixture to a container.

8. e. Add the cucumber, dill, feta, lemon juice, and tomatoes to the couscous, and stir. Pour the couscous mixture into the lamb loin chops and serve.

9. To prepare the lamb loin chops:

10. a. Mix the minced garlic, parsley and salt in a bowl. Put the mixture into the chops by pressing it onto the loin.

11. b. Heat olive oil into a non-stick pan or skilled using from medium to high heat level. Put the lamb loin chops into the hot oil until it is cooked. This will take approximately 10 to 12 minutes.

12. c. Set aside but keep warm.

Ground Round Special a la Turk

4S/LD

Ingredients:

- Quantity   Measure   Food Item
- 1/8   tsp.   Allspice (ground)
- 1/3   cup   Breadcrumbs (dry)
- 1/4   tsp.   Cinnamon (ground) Cooking spray

- 1/2
- tsp.
- Cumin (ground)

- 1 piece Egg (large, beaten lightly)
- 1 tsp. Garlic (used bottled, minced)
- 1 pound Ground round sirloin or any lean beef cut

- 1/4 cup Mint (fresh, chopped)
- 1/2 cup Onion (white, chopped)
- 4 pieces (6 inches) Pita bread (split)
- 2 pieces Plum tomatoes (sliced, 4 to 6 slices per piece)
- 1/4 tsp. Red pepper (ground)
- 1/2 tsp. Salt
- 1 tbsp. Tomato paste
- 1/4 cup Yogurt (low-fat, plain)

Directions:

1. Preheat the broiler in preparation for cooking.

1. Mix the following ingredients in a bowl: allspice, breadcrumbs, cinnamon, cumin, egg, garlic, ground round beef, mint, onion, red pepper, salt, and tomato paste. Stir until the ingredients combine well.

1. Prepare 8 to 12 pieces of patty from the mixture in Step 2.

1. Put cooking spray in a jelly roll pan and place the patties in the oil- coated pan.

1. Broil both sides of the patty for a total of 10 to 15 minutes depending on your preference of how done the patties are.

1. Fill in each half of the pita bread with a patty and a slice of tomato.

1. Garnish each patty-filled pita with yogurt.

1. Relish the goodness of Mediterranean meat cuisine in this ground round special Relish the goodness of Mediterranean meat cuisine in this ground round special

Pasta Rice Bread

Breakfast Rush

5-7   S/BS (Note: When this dish is consumed for snack, the meal plan in Chapter 3 calls it Snack Pack)

Ingredients:

Quantity   Measure   Food Item

- 1   cup   Banana (sliced)
- 1   cup   Granola
- 1   cup   Multigrain cereals

- ½   cup   Raisins
- 1   cup   Rolled oats
- 1   cup   Other fresh or frozen fruit as preferred
- ½   cup   Walnuts or almonds
- 1   cup   Whole grain cereals
- 2   cup   Almond, skim, or soy milk (low-fat)
- 1   cup   Yogurt (plain, low fat or fat-free)

Directions:

1. In a large salad bowl or container (with volume at least 12 cups or 3 liters or 1 gallon, combine the cereals and the oats. If there is no container large enough, divide the ingredients into equal batches of 4.

2. Add the nits and fruits and mix well, but gently.

3. Add in the milk and the yogurt.

4. Pack in smaller containers with cover and store in freezer for no more than 2 days.

Brown Rice Pudding

6S/BS (Note: When this dish is consumed for snack, the meal plan in Chapter 3 calls it Snack Pack)

Ingredients:

- Quantity   Measure   Food Item

- ½   cup   Almonds
- ½   cup   Brown rice
- ½   cup   Butter (low-fat or light)
- ½   tsp.   Cardamom
- 4   cups   Milk
- 1   tbsp.   Orange (zest only)
- ¼   cup   Raisins
- ½   tsp.   Rose water (may not be used if preferred)

Directions:

1. Soak the rice for 10 to 15 minutes in water. Drain

2. Boil the milk and sugar in a sauce pan in medium or high heat to a low boil. Add the cardamom, cinnamon, raisins, and drained rice and bring the mix to a simmer over low heat. Wait for the mixture to thicken before removing from heat. This takes about 45 minutes of simmering with frequent stirring required.

3. Remove from the burner, add the rose water (when preferred).

4. Prepare the almonds and the zest of orange mixture.

5. Use a ladle to transfer the pudding from the pan to serving bowls and top with the almond and orange zest mixture.

6. May be served hot or chilled.

Walnut Baklava

32S/BS

Ingredients:

- Quantity   Measure   Food Item
- ½   cup   Butter (low-fat or light, melted)
- 1   tbsp.   Cardamom
- 2   tbsp.   Cinnamon
- 2   pieces Cinnamon (sticks)
- ½   cup   Honey
- 1   tbsp.   Lemon juice
- 1   tsp.   Lemon (zest)
- ½   cup   Olive oil
- 2   tsp.   Orange (zest)
- ½   pound Phyllo dough (approximately 20 sheets)

- ¼ and 1½   cups   Sugar
- 3   cups   Walnuts
- 1 ½   cup   Water
- 2   cups   Pistachios

Directions:

1. Routine baking preparation procedure: preheat oven to 325 °F.

2. Put cinnamon sticks, honey, lemon juice, 1½ cups sugar, and water in a heavy sauce pan. Boil over medium to high heat for 20 minutes. Remove pan from heat, set aside and cool in the fridge, but remove the cinnamon sticks first.

3. Put the cardamom, cinnamon, the remaining sugar and zests in a food processor and set to course chop (30 pulses).

4. Mix butter and olive oil and brush the mixture on the sides of the baking pan using pantry brush.

5. Unroll the phyllo and cut in halves.

6. Put 1 sheet on the pan, brush with butter-oil mixture and repeat the procedure until all sheets have been brushed.

7. Bake for 1 hours and pour the honey. Set aside for 30 minutes before serving.

8. Poultry

Brown Rice and Stuffed Chicken

10S/LD (Note: Normally served during lunch or dinner, but it's your meal. Nobody will stop you if you want to have it for breakfast.)

Ingredients:

- Quantity   Measure   Food Item
- 2   cups   Chicken stock
- 1   piece   Chicken (whole, weighs approximately 5 pounds, remove giblets)
- 1   piece   Lemon (zest)
- ¼   cup   Olives (green)
- 2   tbsp. and another 1 tbsp.   Olive oil
- 1   piece   Onion (medium sized; chopped)
- 1   tsp.   Paprika
- 1   tsp.   Pepper
- ½   cup   Pine nuts
- 1   cup   Brown rice

- ½ teaspoon Salt
- 2 cups White wine (dry)

Directions:

1. Preheat the oven set to 350 °F.

2. Toss the pine nuts in medium heat for one minute using a 2-quart sauce pan. Add the onions and cook by frequent stirring for 3 minutes.

3. Add the chicken stock and scrape the bottom of the pan to ensure that no nuts stuck.

4. Boil the mixture in medium to high heat. Put the olives and rice, cover the pan and reduce the heat while simmering for about 40 minutes or until the liquid mixture has been absorbed by the rice.

5. Put the chicken in the roast rack of the open. Rub the inside cavity of the chicken with 2 tbsp. of olive oil. Mix in the lemon zest, paprika, pepper, and salt. Rub the spice mixture on the chicken. Brush the chicken with the remaining olive oil.

6. Stuff the chicken with the cooked rice and pour the white wine on the outside part of the chicken.

7. Bake the chicken without cover until the rice and the chicken reach an internal temperature of 165 degrees. Check internal temperature an hour after baking.

8. Baste the chicken every 20 minutes. The baking time is around 1 ½ hours on the average.

9. Set aside the chicken to cool before cutting. Remove the rice from the chicken cavity and transfer into a serving platter.

10. Ideal serving proportion is 2 to 3 ounces of chicken to half cup of rice.

Salad

Greek Salad 4S/BLD

Ingredients:

- Quantity   Measure   Food Item
- 2   pieces Cucumbers (medium-sized; seeded, diced)
- 4   ounces   Feta cheese (crumbled)
- 1   clove   Garlic (minced)
- 1   piece   Lemon (large, juiced)
- ½   cup   Olives (kalamata variety; pitted, chopped)
- 1/3   cup   Olive oil
- ¼   cup   Parsley (fresh, flat leaves, chopped) Pepper (to taste)
- 8   cups   Romaine lettuce (torn into bite size pieces)

- Salt (to taste)
- 4 pieces Tomato (medium sized)

Directions:

1. Put the lettuce in a large salad bowl

2. Cut the tomatoes into 8 wedges each. Place them on top of the lettuce. Add the cucumbers, olives, onions, and parsley.

3. Whisk the following ingredients in a smaller bowl: garlic, lemon juice, and olive oil. Put salt and pepper on the dressing to taste. Pour this in the mixed vegetables from Step 1.

4. Sprinkle with feta cheese and serve immediately.

Snack

- 1 or more S/BS or dessert for a main meal Frutti Smoothies Galore!

- Here are ingredients for a host of Frutti Smoothie snacks which you can prepare beforehand to chill in the freezer. You may also opt to prepare the snack a few minutes before you eat your snack, but for more enjoyable snacking, the ingredients berries, fruit and liquids should be pre-refrigerated. You can prepare a snack of one serving for yourself or multiple servings for your family. Even children love the smoothies!

Ingredients:

1. Berries and Fruits   Liquids   Additional Ingredients
2. Apple sauce Almond milk Apple Almond   butter Granola
3. Blackberries Blueberries   juice Ice   topping Peanut butter
4. Mango   Orange juice Skim milk   Rolled   oats Shredded
5. Peaches   Soy milk   coconut Soy protein
6. Pears Yogurt (low-fat or non-   powder   Whey protein

7. Pineapples Raspberries   fat)   powder

8. Ripe bananas

9. Strawberries

10. Combine your desired ingredients in a quantity that will not make using the blender a challenge. You may get one or more ingredients from each category, but use your imagination to concoct great snack and breakfast ideas.

11. Blend the ingredients until smooth. You may add more ice or liquid as needed.

12. Some smoothie concoctions are shown next page: Frutti Smoothie No. 1

13. Ripe banana Almond milk Rolled oats Almond butter Ice

Frutti Smoothie No. 2

Pineapples Orange juice Granola topping Ice

Frutti Smoothie No. 3

Strawberries Peaches

Skim milk Shredded coconut Ice

Frutti Smoothie No. 4

Apple sauce Apple Juice Yogurt

Rolled oats Ice

Frutti Smoothie No. 5

Blackberries Blueberries Almond milk Yogurt

Whey protein powder Ice

Just keep mixing and matching! Here's Frutti Smoothie No. 3. Yummy!

Soup

Carrot Soup

4S/LD (Note: Normally served during lunch or dinner, but it's your meal. Nobody will stop you if you want to have it for breakfast.)

Ingredients:

- Quantity   Measure   Food Item
- ½   cup   Apple juice (preferably organic)
- 2   pounds   Carrots (preferably organic; peeled and chopped)
- 1 or 2 pinch Curry powder or cumin (better if mild and must be gluten-free)
- 1 or 2 dash Sea salt (to taste, better low sodium for health)

- Water (fresh and cool)

Directions:

1. Put the chopped carrots in a soup pan (pot) and pour enough water to cover the carrots by about an inch.

2. Put a dash of salt and some curry powder or cumin. The amount of curry or cumin depends on you (or your instruction to the person preparing the meal, but normally a pinch or two is enough).

3. Cover the pan (pot) and boil the carrots. After boiling, lower the heat of the burner and allow simmering until the carrots are tender to your desired softness. This should take less than 30 minutes. Add more water if necessary if the initial amount of water is not enough.

4. Turn the soup into a puree using a blender. Stop blending as soon as the carrots are blended and the mixture is smooth.

5. Add the apple juice.

6. A variation to the menu for those who would like to experiment on a creamy one can be made by adding a creamy ingredient such as light coconut milk or the unsweetened type of almond milk instead of apple juice. Other canned cream products may be used depending on your familiarity with the product.

Lentil Soup (Fakkes)

4S/LD (Note: Normally served during lunch or dinner, but it's your meal. Nobody will stop you if you want to have it for breakfast.)

Ingredients:

- Quantity   Measure   Food Item

- 2 pieces Bay leaves
- 1 piece Carrot (medium sized; chopped finely)
- 4 cloves Garlic (whole)
- 1 pound Lentils (dry; this is about 2 cups in volume)
- ½ cup Olive oil (extra virgin)
- 1 piece Onion (medium sized; peeled and grated)
- 1 teaspoon Rosemary (dried)
- 1 cup Tomatoes (fresh or canned; minced and sieved)
  - Water

Directions:

1. Soak the lentils in water overnight.

2. Boil water on a large pot. Rinse the lentils and put them in boiling water for 10 minutes.

3. Drain the water and put in another 6 pints of water and boil.

4. As the mixture boils, add the rest of the ingredients and continue boiling until the lentils are cooked and tender. This usually takes an hour.

5. Remove the bay leaves and serve.

Vegetables

Eggplant and Tomato Pesto

4S/LD (Note: Normally served during lunch or dinner, but it's your meal. Nobody will stop you if you want to have it for breakfast.)

Ingredients:

- Quantity   Measure   Food Item

- 1 cup Basil leaves (add about 15 more leaves for stacking)
  - Cooking spray (non-stick)
- 1 piece Eggplant (sliced round, ½ inch)
- 1 cup Feta cheese (crumbled)
- 1 clove Garlic
- 1 piece Lemon (zest and juice)
- 2 tbsp. Pine nuts
- 2 tbsp. Olive oil
  - Pepper (to taste)

- 2 to 3
- pieces
- Rome tomatoes or beefsteak tomatoes (sliced round, ½ inch)
  - Salt (to taste)
- 1 ½ tsp. Sea salt

Directions:

1. Extract bitterness from the eggplant by rubbing them with salt and topping them with salt afterwards. Set aside for 30 minutes. Rinse afterwards and pat them dry.

1. Blend 1 cup of basil leaves, garlic, lemon juice and zest, olive oil, pine nits, salt, and paper in a blender for 2 to 3 minutes or until the pesto smoothens. Set aside.

1. Spray the eggplant very lightly with the cooking spray. The grill must also be sprayed on.

1. Heat the grill to medium or high heat. Grill both sides of each eggplant round from 3 to 5 minutes or until the desired texture is achieved.
2. Each serving consist of one eggplant round, 1 tsp. of pesto, 1 slice of tomato, and a basil leaf. Top all the garnished eggplants with crumbled feta. Serve.

Bonus - Top Seven Tips for Successful Mediterranean Cooking

Tip No. 1:

Nuts and/or may be sprinkled on breakfast cereal or prepared as homemade spreads, particularly peanuts or tahini. However, if you are using products from the supermarket, read the label to make sure that the sugar and fat content, especially if you are preparing MD recipes for weight loss. Nuts/seeds may also be sprinkled to yogurt for snacks.

Tip No. 2:

Other great uses for nuts and seeds in the kitchen are:

Chopped nuts or seeds are great for bread toppings when baking; Use nuts and seeds for crunchier salads or pasta dishes;

Toast sesame seeds and add these to your stir-fries using healthy nut oils.

Tip No. 3:

Nuts are an everyday staple in the Mediterranean diet as they are used in desserts, salads, and some side dishes. They have to be stored properly so that they will not go rancid. Following are the guidelines for proper storage:

Use glass and plastic containers that are airtight;

Store nuts away from foods with strong odor such as garlic as nuts ted to absorb odor from their surroundings;

Shelled nuts may be kept at room temperature for as long as 3 months and up to 4 months when refrigerated;

Unshelled nuts may last for 4 months when refrigerated and twice as long when kept in the freezer;

If available but nuts from farmers. Otherwise choose to buy nuts from stores that you have observed to have a high turnover rate to ensure freshness;

It is more advisable to buy nuts packaged with a best before or sell-by date to have an idea how long the nuts have been up for sale. Nuts from bins do not in any way guarantee their freshness.

Tip No. 4:

The Mediterranean diet is grounded on the balance of the right foods as reflected in the MD pyramid in Chapter 8. To make the pyramid work for you, consider the following in the preparation of the MD diet:

Fruits and vegetables: Choose by season to ensure freshness
Focus on wholes: Whole grain, whole fruits and vegetables
Fish and shellfish: Best twice per week

Red meat: Small serving once a week

Dairy: Choose only low-fat or fat free and make sure they really are Alcohol: Always consume in moderate amount.

Tip No. 5:

Herbs and spices are a part of Mediterranean cuisine. The following herbs are commonly cultivated in the region: basil, deal, fennel, mint, oregano, parsley, rosemary, sage, and thyme. Feel free to include these in your dishes for that traditional Mediterranean flavor.

Tip No. 6:

Depending on your family's preference, you can tailor your cooking for specific Mediterranean regions. Southern Italian cuisine uses anchovies, balsamic vinegar, basil, bay leaf, capers, garlic, oregano, parsley, peppers, among other herbs and spices. To flavor of the Southern Italian Mediterranean cooking is, therefore zesty with a saucy and spicy hot flavor.

Tip No. 7:

Grecian Mediterranean cuisine has basil, cucumber, dill, fennel, garlic, honey, lemon, mint, olives (of course), oregano, and yogurt. Their flavors therefore run a scale from tangy with citrus accent to savory and bold or soft flavors with creamy texture.

Lightning Source UK Ltd.
Milton Keynes UK
UKHW022110110621
385375UK00002B/230